The Pocket Guide to Grant Applications

A handbook for health care research

Iain K Crombie
Reader in Epidemiology
and
Charles du V Florey
Professor and Head of Department

Department of Epidemiology and Public Health
Dundee University
Ninewells Hospital and Medical School
Dundee

BMJ Books

© BMJ Books 1998
BMJ Books is an imprint of
the BMJ Publishing Group

First published in 1998
by BMJ Books, BMA House, Tavistock Square,
London WC1H 9JR

British Library Cataloguing in Publication Data

A catalogue record for this book is available from the
British Library

ISBN 0-7279-1219-4

Typeset, printed and bound in Great Britain by
Latimer Trend & Company Ltd, Plymouth

The Pocket Guide to Grant Applications

Contents

Chapter 3 Types of grants

Chapter 4 What the grant will cover

Chapter 5 The assessment procedure

Chapter 6 What committees look for

Chapter 7   Common failings

Chapter 8   Strategies for success

Chapter 9   Writing the detailed application

Chapter 10   A computer based aid to writing grants

Preface

This book has been written to help health care researchers write successful grant applications. It is based in part on our experience of preparing grant applications, in which we learned lessons through trial and error. Everyone who submits grant applications encounters rejections and we were no exception. However, we have also had the privilege of sitting on funding committees. This gave us insight into the appraisal criteria that funding committees use and enabled us to identify the characteristics of highly rated applications. This book is an attempt to share this knowledge.

The impetus to write this book came when one of us (IKC) was invited to give a lecture on the appraisal of grant applications from the perspective of a member of a funding committee. This entailed formalising the understanding that had been gained and presenting it in a logical order. Encouraged by the favourable reception the lecture received, we wondered how the information could be shared more widely. This book is the result. It is intended for health professionals and researchers setting out on their grant seeking careers. The text assumes that a good research question has been developed and also that the applicants are familiar with the design and conduct of research studies. In this small book it is not possible to cover how to do research as well as how to write grant applications.

The book chapters fall into three broad sections. Chapters 1–4 review the process of applying for funding and outline the structure of grant applications. The next four chapters describe the main criteria which funding committees use to assess applications, identify the most common pitfalls, and provide a strategy for preparing successful applications. Chapter 9 describes what to include in each section of the grant application and identifies which aspects should be emphasised. The final chapter describes the computer assisted learning package which accompanies the text.

This is on a floppy disk, and is designed to sit on your PC screen alongside the word processing package. It enables the writer to seek advice on the completion of the main sections of the application form. Together, this text and the disk will help the researcher to improve the quality of the grant applications and to increase the likelihood of being funded.

Chapter 1 An overview of the process

Research is as much a feature of today's health service as is the common cold and we are all likely to be exposed to it. The main difference is that research can be useful: it may some day find a cure for the cold. The recent move to research in the NHS was heralded with the launch in 1991 of the Research and Development Initiative. As a result, health professionals are under increased pressure to become involved in research. This is entirely sensible: health professionals have the clinical experience that can give the insights from which good ideas emerge. A major problem they face is that research is time consuming to carry out, and can often only be done when further resources are supplied.

Financial support for research is most readily available in the form of grants from a wide range of funding bodies. Many health professionals have little experience of obtaining these grants. The aim of this chapter is to provide an overview of the process of submitting grant applications, from the initial decision to seek funding through all the stages of the process. The ideas presented briefly in this chapter are developed more fully throughout the rest of the book.

The application process

The writing of a grant application takes place in a series of stages in which the structure and content gradually evolve. The protocol will go through many revisions, as the research question is clarified and details of the research methods are gradually worked out. The several stages are:

- prepare a draft application;
- select the funding body;

- develop the detailed application;
- submit for appraisal;
- await the outcome.

Prepare a draft application

A grant application provides a detailed description of how a study will be conducted. The first draft is written to answer three broad questions.

1. What exactly do we want to find out?
2. Why is it worth finding out?
3. How will we do it?

The purpose of the first draft is to ensure that the proposed research will address a worthwhile question and to encourage discussion of the likely research design. A key part of this is to check that the research is either novel or plans to test a recent and remarkable research claim. The proposed research has to be fitted into the background of what is already known, to clarify the advances which the study will make. A computerised literature search is indispensable for this.

The draft application also tackles the practical issues of what groups of subjects will be studied, what data will be collected, and what resources will be needed to carry out these activities. Writing this draft should identify whether there are major stumbling blocks which could render the project unfeasible. Finally, the first draft should also help clarify which might be the most appropriate funding body.

Select the funding body

There are many funding bodies, each with its own preferences for types of topics and research methods. A project which is of high scientific quality may be turned down by one body, yet welcomed enthusiastically by another. Thus, it is important to match the project to the funding bodies at an early stage. The funding bodies also vary in the size of project they are prepared to fund, making matching more important. Fortunately, many funding bodies welcome informal contacts, at which the suitability of the project can be assessed. Such approaches can yield suggestions to improve the project. They will also identify when a project falls outside the remit of a funding body. The issue of finding a suitable funding body is addressed more fully in Chapter 2.

Develop the detailed application

Funding bodies provide detailed instructions and application forms for the preparation of research protocols. In many instances the application is organised under a similar set of headings. The first, the introduction, gives a brief review of the literature, outlining why new research is needed. The intention is to identify gaps in present knowledge or understanding. Next comes a statement of the study aims or the research questions to be answered. Although short, this is a crucial section of the application. It should follow naturally from the need for the research and should state the aims clearly and succinctly. If the aims are not readily understood by a reviewer, the importance of the research may not be appreciated.

The major part of the grant application gives a full description of the study methods, including the research design to be used, the nature of the subjects to be studied, the data to be collected, and the statistical techniques to be used in the analysis. There are several additional technical requirements such as a financial statement of the resources required together with a justification of these requirements, the CVs of the applicants, and an outline of the potential benefit which will accrue from the research. The application will often run to ten or so pages and may contain 20 or more references.

Although this brief description is far from complete, it serves to make the point that a grant application is a lengthy document and its preparation a major undertaking. This book has been designed to simplify this task.

The structure of the grant application has been designed to elicit information to allow the funding body to decide whether the study is likely to be successful and if it is successful, whether the answers that will be provided will be sufficiently important to merit funding of the study. The importance of following the instructions given by the funding body cannot be stressed strongly enough; if these are ignored, the application may meet immediate rejection. This happens surprisingly often, with predictable consequences.

Submit for appraisal

Most funding bodies have deadlines by which applications must be submitted. Depending on the funding body, this may be only once or up to four times each year. Usually applications have to be submitted at least 6–8 weeks before the meeting of the committee which reviews them. This allows time for the opinions of expert referees to be sought and for the committee members to form their own judgement. It is important not to be late in submitting. Applications received even one day after the deadline can be delayed until the subsequent committee meeting. But while meeting a deadline is important, hastily completed applications should not be submitted. It is usually better to delay until the next round rather than submit a substandard protocol.

Await the outcome

Applications will meet with one of three fates. They can be funded immediately, rejected outright or the applicants may be invited to resubmit. Some projects are funded at first application and these have usually been prepared by experienced researchers. Many applications are rejected at first submission and often these are from inexperienced researchers. Some of these proposals contain good research ideas but are rejected because the application is poorly written or the research methods are incompletely described. They often give the impression that the applicants simply do not understand what is wanted in a proposal and are unaware of the criteria used to evaluate applications. This book has been written to help ensure that this fate is avoided.

Some funding bodies are keen to foster research within the NHS. They may, when presented with a flawed but promising application, invite the applicants to resubmit a revised application. Detailed feedback on any defects, together with suggestions to overcome them, usually accompanies the request for a further submission. There is no guarantee that the revised application will be funded, as it may not be possible to make all the modifications requested by the funding body. However, there is a very good chance of success if close attention is paid to the points raised. The only certainty is that if some of the criticisms are overlooked, the application will be rejected.

The major problems

The major problem in preparing a grant application is finding the time to write it to a high standard. There is little to be said about this other than to recognise it. Only begin if you are sure you will have the time to complete it. There is little point in cobbling together a poor application only to have it rejected.

One consequence of the effort required for preparation is that researchers can be very close to their own projects. They sometimes write them up in a form which appears lucid to them but which may be impenetrable to the external reader. In this case familiarity breeds incomprehension. Applications are much more likely to be funded when ideas and methods are presented in a straightforward logical sequence. This difficulty can be avoided by asking a colleague, or several if possible, to comment on the text. Be attentive to their comments; any misunderstandings are more likely to reflect an opacity of the text than a defect in their intelligence.

The most common reason for applications to be turned down is methodological flaws. The applications are assessed by experts who delight in finding flaws. Thus, the study methods need to be designed and written with great care. If you do not have substantial experience with the chosen research design, some errors may intrude. One recourse is to recruit a more experienced colleague as a mentor. The common failings are reviewed in Chapter 7 and detailed advice on the preparation of the methods section is given in Chapter 9.

The other problem facing those seeking funding is a lack of appreciation of how the application process works. Writing successful grant applications is a craft which has to be learned. Knowing what details to give and what features to emphasise can transform an otherwise dull application into one very likely to be funded. One of the authors of this book had the privilege to work with a scientist who wrote the highest quality applications. He had the gift of presenting the research study he wanted to conduct as if it would provide the major breakthrough which would revolutionise understanding in his field. While few of us have this skill, attention to the advice given throughout this book will help ensure that good ideas are presented in properly prepared applications.

5

Key lessons

Writing a grant application is a time consuming business and should only be undertaken when you are sure you have a good research question. The outcome of any application is uncertain, so it is best to be prepared for rejection. It is vital to prepare the application carefully to maximise the chances of success. The inherent scientific merit of an application is not sufficient to obtain funding. The application must be written to a high standard to meet the criteria applied by funding committees. The rest of this book provides guidance on the preparation of high quality grant applications.

Chapter 2 Where to apply

A common complaint is that there is not as much money around as there used to be. This may be the case, but substantial amounts of research funding are currently available from a diverse range of bodies. These include government institutions, national and local charities, and private companies. Perhaps the real problem is not the overall shortage of funds but a lack of knowledge of the range of funds available. This chapter describes briefly the main sources of funding, giving key addresses so that further information may be obtained.

NHS R&D Initiative

The Department of Health launched the Research and Development initiative for the NHS in April 1991. As part of this initiative, a number of research programmes have been established covering fields such as mental health, cardiovascular disease and stroke, cancer, mother and child health, and asthma. The Health Technology Assessment Programme is one of the largest of these programmes, committing several million pounds to research each year. Within each programme there are calls for applications to conduct research on specific topics, advertised in leading medical journals and in broadsheet newspapers. They are also circulated widely to senior health care staff. The projects range in scale from those for which individuals or small research teams can apply to those conducted using the resources of health authorities or large multicentre, multidisciplinary research groups. The exact procedures vary between programmes and can also change over time. Thus, it is important to obtain up to date details. Useful contact addresses are listed at the end of this chapter, including one for the information pack entitled "Research and Development: towards an evidence-based health service".

Departments of Health

The Departments of Health in England, Scotland, Wales, and Northern Ireland also disburse funds for research. They sometimes commission projects, but will also consider *de novo* applications. The Scots are particularly fortunate in having, through their Chief Scientist Office, substantial funding for medical research. There is some variation between the Departments of Health in their applications procedure. Contact addresses are given at the end of this chapter.

National medical charities

The medical charities play a major role in supporting research. Of these, the largest is the Wellcome Trust with an annual budget of over £150 million. It provides a wide range of types of grants and will consider applications on any topic except AIDS and cancer. Other large charities include the British Heart Foundation, the Arthritis and Rheumatism Council, the National Asthma Campaign, and the National Kidney Research Fund and three cancer charities: the Cancer Research Campaign, the Imperial Cancer Research Fund, and the Leukaemia Research Fund. These charities have annual funds which range from £2 million to £50 million. As their names imply, each of this latter group of charities focuses on a specific disease group. However, all provide many different kinds of grant.

There are a host of other charities, some with substantial sums to disburse (up to £2 million per year), others with smaller amounts (several hundred thousand pounds). Most focus on specific diseases, such as motor neurone disease, Parkinson's disease or brittle bone disease, although some of these smaller national charities have more general remits. They usually fund individual studies although some restrict their awards to specific items such as training, travel or equipment.

Most charities which fund medical research publish annual reports detailing their recent activities and will provide information on application procedures. The addresses of these charities, together with details of the types of research which they fund, are listed in the *Association of Medical Research Charities Handbook*, copies of which can be obtained from the address at the end of this chapter.

Medical Research Council

The Medical Research Council (MRC) is a leading funding body, supporting research across the whole range of medicine from fundamental molecular biology through to health services research. It has a total budget in excess of £300 million. The MRC provides a wide range of types of grants including training fellowships and travel grants and further information can be obtained from the address given at the end of this chapter. The structure for supporting research was revised in 1997, placing increasing emphasis on large scale, multidisciplinary research where applications are prepared by high calibre collaborative teams, often based in more than one institution. However, there are also proposals to establish grants for newly appointed university scientists as well as innovation grants to provide short term funding for high risk or speculative research.

The MRC publishes a handbook which describes the features and functioning of the MRC and an annual report which outlines recent progress in research and indicates priorities for the future. Details of the types of grants available are routinely circulated and are available on request. Particular prestige attaches to gaining a grant from the MRC and competition for them is fierce. Only applications of the highest quality will be funded.

Local sources

Many regions have local charities which fund research and most hospital trusts have their own research funds. Most trusts will also have a research and development lead officer, one of whose tasks is to compile data on all available funding bodies. Health authorities have research managers who fulfil a similar role. These individuals will be be able to supply details of the local as well as the national funding sources.

The attraction of local funding sources is that they naturally look kindly on local applicants. Often the application procedures are more informal (although seldom less rigorous). This may give greater opportunities to discuss and modify the application to fit more closely with the expectations of the local funding body.

Other sources

There are many other sources of research funds. The most wealthy of these is the European Commission which supports biomedical and health research with a budget of over £150 million. Its projects must involve two, or preferably more, member countries of the European Union. The funding process is complex and protracted and it is recommended that the services of a specialist adviser be obtained. Only experienced researchers should consider applying for these funds.

Funding is also available from the European Science Foundation (ESF), a body unrelated to the European Commission. This is an independent association of research councils, academies and institutions; the MRC is one of the UK members. The ESF is particularly concerned with the exchange of information and ideas between research teams across member countries. It funds a range of activities including conferences, workshops, and networks.

The Economic and Social Research Council (ESRC) is a comparable organisation to the Medical Research Council (MRC). The ESRC funds studies which are primarily sociological, psychological or economic but will consider those which have a medical component. If it considers that an application is primarily medical it will pass it to the MRC.

Many professional societies have some funds available for research. These include the colleges of nursing and midwifery as well as many of the medical colleges. Even if they do not have funds they may well know of funds which are earmarked for your profession. Thus it is well worth approaching your professional society for advice about funding.

Most of the major drug companies and some of the medical equipment manufacturers sponsor medical research. Sometimes this can be related to the development and marketing of their products but a substantial amount of money is distributed as part of a more general policy of fostering the development of medicine. The problem with obtaining drug company sponsorship is knowing how to apply. Sometimes adverts inviting submissions will appear in medical journals. More often, submissions will be made when there is a good working relationship between a health care professional and a drug company. The researcher knows the types of topic the company might be interested in and can discuss preliminary ideas with them. The company knows the researcher and will be confident that high quality research will be carried out. The only way into this source of funding is to cultivate contacts with the companies, a strategy for the long rather than the short term.

Key lessons

This chapter has reviewed the diversity of the organisations which fund medical research. They vary in the sums of money they disburse, the types of grant they award, and the topics they prefer to fund. It is not possible to provide comprehensive coverage of all possible funding sources here as the available information would require at least a book to itself. The key lesson is that there are lots of them out there and a small investment of time to try to identify those which may fund your type of research is well worthwhile. Trying to cover all the funding bodies at once would consume so much time and energy that none would be left for writing the application. It would be better to adopt a sequential approach starting with a few funding bodies, possibly those from whom colleagues have gained support. Then the field could be gradually expanded as need and time permit.

There are several sources of information on funding bodies. All funding bodies provide instructions to applicants, which review their research interests and outline the application procedures. Most also produce annual reports which detail current and completed projects so you can check whether your study fits in with the general run of funded studies. These annual reports will usually also describe any recent changes to research priorities. Many funding bodies also welcome informal approaches from potential applicants, to discuss the submission process and the details of the specific application. But one word of caution. Whatever the source of the information or advice, make sure that you take it. If funding bodies have taken pains to supply detailed information, it would be churlish to ignore it.

Websites

Substantial amounts of information are now available on the Internet, addresses for which are listed below. One of the most useful is the Wisdom Schemes Search produced by the Wellcome Trust. This contains over 300 funding sources which users can search by subject area, type of award, and key words. The information contained in the *Association of Medical Research Charities Handbook* is also available on the Internet. It can be searched by type of grant and through an alphabetical listing of the charities. Finally, extensive information is available on the NHS R&D Initiative. This information is spread across several sites and three addresses are given below to help users access these sites.

Wisdom Schemes Search (Wellcome Trust)
   http://wisdom.wellcome.ac.uk/wisdom/schemes.html

Association of Medical Research Charities
   http://www.amrc.org.uk/homepage.htm

NHS National R&D information
   http://libsun1.jr2.ox.ac.uk:80/nhserdd/national.htm

NHS National Priority Research Programmes
   http://libsun1.jr2.ox.ac.uk:80/nhserdd/aordd/overview/
   commr&d.htm

NHS Technology Assessment Programme
   http://www.soton.ac.uk/ ~ wi/hta

Contact addresses

NHS R&D Initiative
Office of the Director of the Research and Development
Department of Health
Richmond House
79 Whitehall
London   Fax: 0171 210 5868

Copies of the information pack entitled "Research and Development: towards an evidence-based health service" can be obtained from:

Research and Development Division
Room 402A
Skipton House
80 London Road
London SE1 6LW

Health Technology Assessment Programme
HTA Programme Manager
Research and Development Directorate
NHS Executive
Room GW52, Quarry House
Quarry Hill   Tel: 0113 254 6194
Leeds LS2 7UE   Fax: 0113 254 6174/6197

Department of Health
Room 449
Richmond House
79 Whitehall
London SW1A 2NS

Scottish Office Department of Health
Chief Scientist Office
St Andrew's House   Tel: 0131 244 2244
Edinburgh EH1 3DG   Fax: 0131 244 2683

The Association of Medical Research Charities
29–35 Farringdon Road
London EC1M 3JB

The Medical Research Council
20 Park Crescent
London W1N 4AL   Tel: 0171 636 5422

Economic and Social Research Council
Polaris House
North Star Avenue   Tel: 01793 413000
Swindon SN2 1UJ   Fax: 01793 413001

European Science Foundation
1 quai Lezay-Marnesia
67080 Strasbourg   Tel: 00 3 33 88 76 71 00
France   Fax: 00 3 33 88 37 05 32

Chapter 3 Types of grants

There are many different types of grant for which submissions may be made. They provide sums of money which range from a few hundred pounds to many hundreds of thousand pounds. They also differ in their intentions: many provide full support for a single research study; some provide support for development or pilot work; others have a staff training element. This chapter reviews these various types of grants to assist researchers in identifying the one which best meets their funding needs.

Project grants

The most common type of grant is, as the name implies, one designed to support the conduct of a specific project. All the major funding bodies, except the MRC, award project grants and the main business of grants committees is deciding which of the many project grant applications they receive should be awarded funding. These grants often cover the salary of a full time research assistant for two or three years together with any costs encountered in conducting the research. However, there are many opportunities to seek smaller sums to conduct smaller scale research studies. Whatever their size, project grants are the ones for which most researchers should be aiming. The main focus of this book concerns the design of successful project grant applications.

Programme grants

Programme grants supply substantial funding, upwards of £500 000, to conduct a large scale study or a series of closely related research studies. They often support a research team of one or two research fellows and two or three support staff, as well as providing equipment and running costs. It would be wonderful to gain such a grant, but so would it be to find the pot of gold at the end of the rainbow. Only a few of these grants are awarded and they are only given to researchers with international reputations. Funding bodies will only risk such large sums of money to experienced researchers who have proven they have the vision and the ability to conduct groundbreaking research. Getting such a grant could be a long term career ambition but for most researchers it is not to be pursued in the immediate future.

Training fellowships

Many health professionals wish to develop their research skills but find that the lack of time and opportunity are major barriers. Yet it is recognised that medical research needs health professionals who are active in research: it is from the insights gained in routine practice that many important research questions are identified. To enable health professionals to develop the necessary expertise, training fellowships were established. They provide funding for the secondment of health care staff, either full or part time, for periods of between one and four years. Funding bodies vary in the types of training fellowships which they offer, both in duration and in the proportion of time spent in training. Commonly, suitable candidates identified from written applications are invited for interview. This will cover the proposed research and the benefits which the candidate will gain from it.

The main requirements for fellowship funding are that an appropriate training programme must be identified and there must be a well defined project on which the applicant would work. The training programme should be fitted to the trainee's needs, providing expertise as required on research design, statistics, computing, economics or qualitative methods. The research project should also be geared to assist the professional development of the trainee. Funding committees are primarily concerned with what the trainee will gain from the fellowship. Thus, there will be little support for a project in which the trainee is simply a pair of hands providing technical assistance.

Training fellowships are commonly based in a university department, which will provide supervision and contribute to the training programme. It is remarkably easy to find a university department which will play the host role. Universities are under increasing pressure to bring in research grants and would look more than kindly at someone who offered to bring one with them. The training element is easily arranged by enrolling the applicant to take modules from existing postgraduate courses. If you wish to apply for one of these fellowships, it is best to contact a university department at an early stage, to benefit from their experience in submitting applications.

Mini grants

Mini grants, or small project grants, were established to provide small sums of money more speedily than is the case for larger project grants. The sums involved range from a few hundred pounds up to £25 000. The mini project grant is assessed quickly and the award can be made within a few weeks of submission. This compares with 3–6 months (and sometimes longer) for conventional project grants. As well as funding small scale projects, these grants are intended to support development or pilot work which can precede a much larger study.

Mini grants provide an attractive option for researchers, but do not be fooled into thinking that they are a soft option. These grants are subject to a thorough appraisal by external referees and by the professional staff of the funding body. Although the scale of the research may be less than a full project grant, broadly similar criteria are used to decide whether to grant funding. Thus, mini grants need to be prepared with the same rigour as larger project grants and need to be carefully written because, as they are shorter, there is less space in which to describe the research.

Calls for proposals

Many funding bodies issue calls for applications on selected topics. This is the sole way in which the Health Technology Assessment Programme operates. Other bodies, such as the MRC or the Chief

17

Scientist Office, issue intermittent calls for proposals on topics of immediate concern. For example, the Gulf War syndrome generated sufficient concern to provoke a request for applications to investigate it. Calls are also issued for research in broad areas. For example, there have recently been calls for studies on mental health and on health services research. These have the twin aims of conducting specific research projects and of fostering research within these broad areas.

Calls for proposals appear attractive to researchers. They provide a stimulus to write and a deadline for submission. This type of grant automatically overcomes one of the major hurdles to funding: being of interest to the funding body. Sometimes projects may be methodologically sound but will meet with rejection because they do not attract the interest of the funding body. Submission in response to a call means this will not happen.

The advantage of calls for applications will only hold when your project's aims will answer in full the research questions given in the call. It may seem surprising but as many as 50% of applications will be rejected immediately because they do not meet the requirements expressed in the call. Some applicants appear to think it is worth submitting projects that fall within the same general area as that covered by the call. This is not the case. Calls for applications are issued when a funding body wants answers to some specific research questions. Projects tackling related areas will be of little interest.

The drawback with calls for proposals is that they will generate several, possibly as many as 30, submissions on each topic. Thus your application is in competition with others. Unlike other funding approaches, where an application stands or falls on its own merits, competition can result in a good application failing because it comes up against one that is truly excellent. This is likely to be the case when the topic of the call is one in which you have some interest but are not an expert. Your application is likely to be in competition with others from experts in the field. Inevitably their applications will be of higher quality than your own. Because of the uncertainty surrounding the competition, some researchers only respond to calls on topics on which they had previously planned to make a submission.

Other types of grants

Some funding bodies take an active role in fostering contact and collaboration between scientists. They will pay for travel to other countries, together with reasonable subsistence costs while staying there, so that researchers can gain experience of the techniques and research strategies. It can be easier to gain funding if the research group you wish to visit has an international reputation. Fortunately, these research groups often welcome visitors who come with funding and with ideas for collaborative research. To gain the funding, you need to be able to make a good case for the benefits you will gain from the visit.

Scientific meetings, symposia or workshops play an important role in the dissemination of findings and the generation of new research ideas. This value is recognised by several funding bodies who in consequence will provide some financial support. Often the support is not given to meetings organised by established learned societies as they are considered to be capable of generating sufficient funds themselves.

Some funding bodies offer senior research fellowships which can be accompanied with a personal chair. These are for experienced researchers who, because they do not have a permanent post, need funding to continue their research. These applications are normally supported by the host institution in which the researcher will work.

Researchers are sometimes impeded in their research because they lack some specialist piece of equipment. The equipment may not be needed solely for a single project, but could facilitate a range of projects. Many funding bodies have specific applications procedures for obtaining equipment.

Two stage applications

Sometimes funding bodies institute a two stage application process. This is the standard approach for the Health Technology Assessment Programme, the Wellcome Trust, and some of the other charities. At the first stage an outline of the project is submitted, giving a brief introduction, a statement of the aims of the research, and a summary of the methods. If the proposal is thought likely to be funded, the applicants are requested to submit

19

a more detailed application. This is an attractive process for researchers because of the smaller investment in preparing the initial application. It is better to be turned down at this early stage than to labour over the full application only to have it rejected.

The preliminary application will often be no more than one or two pages of A4 paper. (It is essential not to exceed the stated length as doing so can lead to summary rejection.) The brief details allow the funding body to decide whether the topic is of interest, whether the project appears feasible, and whether the applicants have sufficient experience to be able to carry it out. The space limitations mean that a detailed explanation of the method cannot be given. Nonetheless, vague general descriptions should be avoided. Instead, try to give the essential study details: the research method, the characteristics and the number of study subjects, the measurements to be made, the statistical techniques to be used. Finally, make sure you request sufficient resources at the first application. It will be difficult if later, when preparing the full application, you discover that more is needed than was first thought.

Key lessons

This chapter has explored the variety of grants. Researchers can match the scale of their project and its detailed requirements to the most appropriate type of grant. The commonest type of grant is the project grant. Most researchers begin their careers by applying for this type of grant. The rest of this book focuses on how to write high quality project grants. However, the principles which lie behind the advice given apply to all types of grant.

Chapter 4 What the grant will cover

A question often faced by researchers applying for their first research grant is "What can I claim for?". The simple answer is that research grants will normally cover all the extra costs which arise during the conduct of the study. This includes the research staff who may be needed to help in the study, essential equipment, and running costs such as postage, travel, and photocopying. This chapter reviews the types of items which can be included under each of these headings.

Research staff

It is recognised that full time health professionals, or even academics for that matter, do not have time to carry out all the tasks of a research project themselves. Instead, they are expected to provide adequate supervision of research staff funded by the project grant. (Providing this supervision is essential, normally amounting to several hours, at least four, of dedicated time each week.) The choice of staff will reflect the skills needed to carry out the research, but will often involve graduates in an appropriate specialty (e.g. statistics, psychology or economics) or a suitably qualified health professional (e.g. nurse, laboratory technician or physiotherapist). It is easiest to get funding if only one research associate is requested. More than one will invite suspicion, unless the project is a large multicentre study tackling a question of major importance. However, support for a secretary, often only part time, can also be claimed if there are many clerical duties to be performed (such as scheduling patient appointments, typing invitation letters or dealing with telephone enquiries).

As well as the type of staff, there is the question of the level at which they should be appointed. The adage "*If you pay peanuts you get monkeys*" applies with as much force in research as elsewhere. Make sure you appoint someone with adequate skills: if a novice is appointed to a demanding post the supervisor will end up doing much of the work. Funding bodies will usually accept a cogent argument for an experienced research assistant. Certainly they expect that a substantial proportion of the total costs will be for staff.

Most staff will be on incremental pay scales and allowance must be made for this when budgeting: a research assistant may earn more than £1000 extra at the end of the study than at the beginning. National pay awards are a different matter; as they cannot be predicted, they are not really the responsibility of the applicants. Most funding bodies will honour these awards, although it is worth checking if you are in doubt. Some of the smaller funding bodies may not make provision for this.

Essential equipment

Research studies can have very diverse needs for equipment. They may need peak flow meters to measure respiratory function, tape recorders to record conversations or dipsticks to measure urine glucose. Funding for all of these can be requested. Any item which would not normally be available, or is required in quantities which would not be available, can be claimed.

Most studies collect large amounts of data so that a computer will be required for the analysis. This, together with necessary software, can be claimed. A good quality printer will also be needed to write letters, print questionnaires, and prepare reports. However, sophisticated top of the range machines or colour laser printers will seldom be justified.

Running costs

Research studies encounter many day to day running costs. Common ones are postage, stationery, photocopying, interlibrary loans, preparation of slides for conference presentations, computer supplies (disks, toner). Some of these items may seem trivial but if they are not claimed for under the grant, some other source of funding will be needed. The researcher needs to envisage all contingencies and to budget accordingly.

Travel and subsistence

Projects which involve travel to distant sites, to access records or to conduct interviews, can apply for appropriate expenses. The researcher's host institutions will have set rates for travel and subsistence, which the funding body will be happy to meet. You should not expect to live in luxury whilst travelling, but nor should you have to survive in penury.

Trips to exotic locations are generally frowned upon, unless the trip is to present the findings of the research to a scientific meeting. This latter is a legitimate expense, and some funding bodies introduce an element into their award to cover such trips. Other funding bodies request separate applications for conference travel, and must be persuaded that the expense is justified.

An average grant

To show how the various costs come together, a budget has been prepared for a hypothetical study (Table 4.1). The project would be considered modest by some of the major funding bodies although it would stretch the limits of others. This project is to investigate the experiences of patients following day case surgery, there being concerns that some patients suffer some distress (pain and nausea) in the first few days following discharge. The study would involve home interviews with patients to ascertain their experiences and determine their use of other services (e.g. the GP). The interviews would be carried out by a nurse who had experience of research and interviewing. Thus, a G grade nurse would be required. The study would involve about 150 patients (a statistician has estimated the required sample size) and the project will take 18 months to complete. To process and analyse the data, a computer and associated software will be required. A variety of running costs will be encountered and these will be higher in the first year of the

TABLE 4.1 *Costings for a project grant*

	Year 1 £	Year 2 £	Year 3 £	Total £
(a) Staff salaries:				
Research assistant 1B				
(point 15)	23 233	12 066		
Employer's costs	6041	3137		
Subtotal	29 274	15 203		44 477
45% overhead	13 173	6841		
Subtotal (a)				**64 491**
(b) Equipment (inc VAT if applicable)				
Viglen Genie pci				
p5/150 computer	1129			
Hewlett Packard				
Deskjet printer	300			
Software (Microsoft Office Professional, SPSS for Windows,				
Nud*ist)	550			
Subtotal (b)	**1979**			**1979**
(c) Consumables				
Computer consumables	100	50		
Postage	250	100		
Stationery	300	100		
Office consumables	150	50		
Photocopying	400	100		
Interlibrary loans	100	100		
Subtotal (c)	**1300**	**500**		**1800**
(d) Other expenses (please specify)				
Travel	4000			
Subsistence while				
travelling	800	200		
Data entry/ secretarial	900	400		
Subtotal (d)	**5700**	**600**		**6300**
Totals	44 108	19 344		74 570

project. Finally, because the project involves home visits, there will be quite substantial travelling and subsistence costs.

Table 4.1 shows the costs for the various items laid out in a form commonly employed in grant applications. The salary is stated year by year, giving the employer's costs separately. Large items of equipment are listed individually, whereas smaller items are given as groupings of consumables. The working rule is to give as much detail as possible without being tiresome. Committees are unwilling to award thousands of pounds without some explanation, but items which cost only a few pounds can be grouped under a more general heading.

One entry in Table 4.1 which might need some explanation is the 45% overhead on salary. This item is only payable when the applicants are based in a university. It is intended to cover some of the institutional costs such as office space, heating and lighting, the library, and information technology support services. The overhead is only paid by some of the funding bodies, particularly the research councils and government sponsored research. Medical charities do not pay it. Finance officers will be able to advise when the overhead should be included.

Key lessons

Funding bodies have substantial experience with the costs of research and will happily meet all reasonable expenses. Resource requirements need to be planned carefully. The costing should be realistic to achieve your aims. It is best not to try to cut corners to reduce costs. Funding bodies are interested in high quality research and will pay a little extra to get it. Perhaps the worst outcome is to underestimate the requirements so that the project comes unstuck when it is almost finished. Some funding bodies will bail a project out but if the overspend was in the least predictable, questions will be raised about the competence of the applicants. This could prejudice subsequent applications.

Although funding bodies will generally award the resources which are really needed for a project, make sure that all items are properly justified. There is little that gives a committee member more pleasure than spotting excessive staff time or self-indulgent luxury items. More importantly, applying for inappropriate resources can create the impression that the applicants do not really know what they are about. Such an impression will harm the chances of funding. Better to check the details, asking of each one whether it is necessary.

Chapter 5 The assessment procedure

Grant applications are assessed by several groups of individuals. These include expert referees, the professional staff of the funding body, and a formal grants committee comprising senior health professionals and academics. These individuals have differing, if sometimes overlapping, perspectives and together their appraisal is detailed and thorough. This chapter explores the roles and perspectives of the groups involved in the assessment of grant applications.

External referees

Grant applications are sent for review to external referees, usually at least two, sometimes as many as four, and occasionally as many as seven or eight. They are chosen for their expertise on the particular research topic and will generally have substantial research experience. Some funding bodies ask the applicants to nominate a referee. This enables experienced researchers to put forward a friend. If you can't do this, try to pick someone with experience of the type of study you want to do. Such people are more likely to be sympathetic to the problems of conducting the research.

Because of their expert knowledge, referees will indicate whether the research is novel and whether it will make a substantial contribution to knowledge. The referees will often have conducted similar research studies to the one proposed so can comment on its feasibility. They will inspect the design carefully for flaws which could invalidate any findings. The views of the external referees are given in writing and presented to the grants committee by the professional secretary.

The referees' views represent an individual opinion and inevitably there will be differences between individuals. Some may rate a project highly because it fits with a personal view of how research in the field should be pursued. Others may rate the same project poorly because they think the topic dull or consider the methods inherently flawed. It is because of this potential for diversity of view that several referees are approached. From their combined opinions, salient points are sought about originality and the existence of flaws.

The funding body's view

Funding bodies, like any institution or private company, have mission statements which include lists of their research priorities. Thus, when reviewing the intrinsic merits of an application, the funding body will rate the priority of the topic. This will lead some proposals to be rejected immediately as being beyond the purview of the organisation. Other proposals may be carried forward only to be rejected later because of a modest priority rating. The ideal strategy is to target grant applications to a carefully selected funding body so that they can benefit from a high priority grade.

The committee's assessment

The committees which assess and vote on grant applications often comprise 15–20 people. They are chosen to cover a range of academic disciplines (several medical specialties as well as psychology, economics, statistics, and sociology). There may also be representatives of many branches of the health service, including management and nursing. Some committees may also have lay members. Together, the committee will have a breadth of specialist knowledge and substantial research experience. It will also be abreast of current medical, social, and political developments.

Many committees function in broadly the same way. A critique of each application is presented to the whole committee by two of its members, often termed the lead and the second speaker. They will have read the application with care, assessing it on the criteria outlined in Chapter 7. The views of the two speakers have a powerful influence on the decisions the committee takes. Other members of the committee will have briefly inspected the applications, giving more time to those which fall in their field of interest. (It is not possible for all committee members to read each application in depth; there may be between 15 and 30 applications to review and each will take at least two hours to assess properly.) The discussions which follow the speakers' presentations can be lively. Committee members take account of referees' and speakers' opinions but often voice strongly held personal views. Comments can range from "poorly designed inconsequential data grabbing" to "very well written protocol of great importance which must be funded".

Making the decision

After a period of discussion the chairman will summarise the views which have been expressed, indicating where there is a consensus. The committee members then assign a score. The scoring is private to allow individuals to express their views without fear of comment from others. Projects with the highest average scores are funded first, moving down the ranks of progressively lower scoring applications until the available monies are committed. It is usually not necessary to assign a minimum level for funding as the money will all be allocated well before a minimum score is encountered.

Key lessons

This chapter has described how thorough an appraisal each application receives. There is such a breadth of committee expertise that failings will commonly be exposed. The process, involving so many individuals, is broadly fair although in the nature of human frailty, mistakes may be made. Some projects are rejected because they are assessed as being of low priority by the grants committee but most unsuccessful applications are rejected because they fail to meet one or more of the appraisal criteria applied by funding committees. These criteria are reviewed in the next chapter.

Chapter 6 What committees look for

Grant applications need to be written to meet the appraisal criteria of funding committees. Many funding bodies issue guidelines, sometimes in the form of a series of questions, which committee members can use to assess grant applications. Rather than reproduce overlapping sets of items, this chapter presents the criteria common to all funding bodies.

An important research question

It is natural that funding bodies wish to support important research. They want to make the best use of their resources and contribute to the discoveries that transform the delivery of health care. Thus, the importance of the research question needs to be stressed in the application. It is not enough to have a research question which strikes the researcher as important. The reasons need to be apparent to even a cursory inspection of the application. Some application forms have a section entitled "The need for further research". Even if this is not asked, it is an excellent practice to provide it. Then even the most obtuse of committee members should appreciate the value of the research.

There are many factors which contribute to the importance of research, centring on the potential to reduce human suffering. This could either be the development of new forms of treatments or new methods of providing care. Or it could be in terms of theoretical understanding of the causation or progress of disease. Finally, it could be research which provides insights into the operation of the NHS, the processes which influence decision making or the factors which determine professional or patient behaviour. These diverse topics have a common feature; that research findings from them will be generalisable across the whole of the country.

The type of disease will also influence importance. Thus, a major advance in a minor disease or a more modest advance in a major disease would count as important. Major diseases are those which cause either death, suffering and disability or which result in substantial cost to the NHS. This is why conditions such as heart disease and cancer attract very large amounts of research money whereas others, such as dandruff and acne, are largely ignored.

A timely topic

As part of their preparation for writing this book, the authors took careful note of the types of projects funded by the committees on which they sat. By far the most prominent feature of successful applications was timeliness of the topic. There were many examples of this. Some applications picked up on authoritative guidelines issued by a learned medical body. The projects addressed the extent to which the guidelines were implemented, the barriers to their implementation or sought to test new methods to encourage their implementation. Other applications focused on issues which had recently been highlighted in editorials in leading medical journals. Yet others were on topics which had been listed as strategic health care targets in the *Health of the Nation* report. Finally, some applications concentrated on issues arising from the use of recently developed technologies such as genetic engineering and minimal access surgery. A common theme to these projects is that there is an opportunity which, if not taken now, may be lost. Funding committees are sensitive to this argument.

Timeliness can be a powerful factor for another reason. Topics which have been recently raised are at once familiar to the funding committee and carry the cachet of the professional group which raised them. There is an unstated assumption that current issues are inherently more interesting than past ones. Past issues may not have been adequately addressed and the requisite research may never have been conducted. Nonetheless, studies to investigate them may be thought dull in comparison with those on topics which are current. There is little point in railing against fashion in research; it is not a policy of funding bodies to be fashionable. Instead, the researcher should take advantage of timely events where possible. If this is not possible then the extra difficulty of

31

gaining funding for non-topical subjects should be recognised. Additional efforts need to be made to stress the importance of the research question, the need for further research, and the potential implications of the study.

A well presented application

It might not be thought that committees would pay overmuch attention to the appearance of an application. It is true that appearance need not equate with content but a shabby looking application gives the impression that it has been cobbled together. By implication, the study methods may not have been adequately worked out. In contrast, a well laid out, neatly typed application suggests attention to detail, which bodes well for the research design. No matter how objectively an application is assessed, there is always a subjective element when it comes to scoring. The overall impression created by the application could tip the balance for or against funding.

But there is another reason for improving the looks of an application. Funding committees have many applications to review and its members become tired as they work steadily through them. If an application is cluttered or poorly laid out, one or more of the key details may be misunderstood. The study may be considered flawed and thus rejected. This may be unfortunate, but is understandable. Committee members are human too and make mistakes like everyone else. Thus, it is best to minimise the risk by constructing well presented applications.

An appropriate research method

There is a variety of research methods including clinical trials, case series, cross-sectional surveys, cohort studies, and case control studies as well as many forms of qualitative methods. Each has its place, being better suited to some research questions than to others. Thus, to assess the effectiveness of a treatment, the recognised method is the clinical trial. The natural history of a disease is best covered with a cohort study. Rare adverse drug reactions can be investigated either by a case control study or a cohort study (the choice will be influenced by the characteristics of the drug and the nature of the adverse reaction). Funding committees recognise this diversity among research methods. They will therefore ask whether the chosen method is the most suitable for the stated research question. The books listed at the end of this chapter provide guidance on matching research questions with methods.

Methodological rigour

Every research method has a set of key steps which must be covered in the description of the study design. Further, every method has its recognised pitfalls, the stages at which things can go seriously wrong. For example, in a clinical trial the key steps are defining and recruiting the patient group, randomisation, preservation of blindness, and the assessment of outcome. Pitfalls include poor compliance and the loss of patients to follow up.

The characteristics of the common research methods are well known to funding committees who expect them to be fully covered in the description of the research design. The key steps of the main research methods are listed at the end of this chapter, outlining the key features of research studies. Referral to these will help ensure that the requisite steps have been covered.

The requirement to fund only high quality studies means that committees naturally adopt a sceptical approach to appraising grant applications. There is almost a presumption that a protocol will be flawed and it is just a matter of finding out where. To deny the committee the pleasure of finding the flaws, you should search for them yourself. Act as a devil's advocate and ask questions such as:

- Will the method of recruiting patients result in an atypical group?
- Will some groups of patients be more likely to respond than others?
- Could knowledge that they are taking part in a study influence behaviour?
- During the study, are certain types of patients (e.g. healthy ones or very sick ones) likely to disappear from view?
- Will the person doing the data collection receive adequate training?

- If more than one person collects data, will the measurements be standardised?

If you identify instances where bias could creep in, then the design should been modified to preclude this. When this has been done, it is worth describing briefly the improvements that have been made to the study. This will show that careful thought has been given to the design. However, don't overdo the description of potential flaws as this could give quite the wrong impression.

Feasibility

The method may be perfectly worked out, but this does not guarantee that it will work in practice. A number of additional questions will be asked:

- Can enough patients be recruited?
- Will cooperation be forthcoming from the professional groups involved?
- Can accurate data be collected?
- Can the study be achieved in the time stated given the available resources?

Every stage of the project should be thought through, seeking an answer to the question: "Where might it go wrong?". Thus the grant application should anticipate the searching questions and provide explicit answers so that reassurance will be found. For example, it helps to state why sufficient patients will be recruited (e.g. because many more than this are seen in a typical year). It also helps to cite references which confirm the validity and reliability of the data collection methods. Mentioning pilot work which has demonstrated the feasibility of parts of the study can greatly strengthen an application. Finally, the major milestones should be presented in a timetable, showing, for example, how long the pilot study will take, when patient recruitment will start and stop. This will help the researcher and the funding committee decide whether the study can be completed in the allotted time. It also provides a convenient method to monitor study progress.

Experienced researchers

Funding bodies are more confident about giving out money when the recipients have a track record of successful research. It is an axiom of psychology that the best predictor of future behaviour is past behaviour. Equally in research, those who have carried out high quality work in the past are a good bet for doing so in the future. The closer the field of the past research is to the new proposal, the stronger this relationship is deemed to be. Funding bodies are also concerned that researchers have sufficient permanence of appointment to see the project to completion.

Grant applications request the CVs of applicants and these are studied carefully to ensure that they demonstrate the necessary skills. The CVs are brief and need to be carefully written, listing job title and papers published, to give the sought after reassurance.

This emphasis on past success presents something of a problem to new researchers and to those who wish to undertake research in a new field. While understanding funding bodies' reluctance to take risks, it seems unfair that junior staff are unable to break in to the system. The exception to this is when junior staff have more experienced researchers as collaborators. Funding committees may then be favourably disposed to giving the junior researcher a leg up. The committee will rely on the experienced collaborator to teach and guide, to ensure the study is successfully completed. The problem is that it can be difficult to find such support. Experienced researchers usually have their own research portfolio and may be unwilling to take on someone else's project. Then again, the kudos of helping bring in another grant, at the price of providing some supervision, will often win them over. It is well worth the effort of trying to recruit an experienced co-applicant: unsupported junior staff will find it difficult to gain funding.

Implications of the findings

The part of the grant application which often receives least attention is the implications which flow from the findings of the study. Even if all other parts are excellent, the application will not be funded if the implications are not clearly spelled out.

One of the weakest statements of implications is to identify further research which could be stimulated by the study. Research commonly begets research and it would be surprising if no further studies could be identified. Instead, more positive benefits need to be identified. One way of achieving this is to try to answer the following questions:

- Who will be directly affected by the findings (which patient groups and which health professionals)?
- What changes in health care delivery might follow from a successful study? How much improvement in health could be obtained?
- How does the research fit in with national priorities?
- Could the study lead to reductions in health service use or other types of cost savings?
- What contribution to fundamental knowledge comes from the study?
- Are there general principles underlying the findings which have implications for other groups of patients?
- Could the findings have implications for postgraduate medical education?
- Which professional groups could benefit from the findings?

The potential implications need to be written with the funding body in mind. For example, the medical charities will be particularly interested in improvements in patient care and well being. However, to the Department of Health, cost savings would be equally important, since any monies saved could be diverted elsewhere.

Dissemination

Funding bodies are placing increasing emphasis on the dissemination of study findings. Some grant applications ask explicitly for this but even if they do not, the issue should be covered. Getting research into practice is a buzz phrase for the NHS in the 1990s. It is not enough to say the findings will be presented at scientific meetings and published in medical journals. This is expected of all studies. More impressive is to identify key organisations and professional societies who would be informed of the findings. It can also help to mention the local groups who will be contacted. Some research groups disseminate their findings by holding regional workshops. The costs of organising these can be included in the costings for the study. The idea is to demonstrate that thought has been given and that effort will be put into the dissemination of the results.

Key lessons

Funding committees ask three general questions of research proposals:

1. Will the study succeed?
2. Will the answer be worth having?
3. Does the study represent value for money?

The grant application must make clear that the answer to all three is a resounding yes. Thus, the application must be clearly written and free from ambiguity. The research method should be appropriate for the research question and the description of the method should provide sufficient detail to convince the reviewer that the study will succeed. Finally, a good case should be made for why the research is necessary and why the findings will have wide reaching implications. The application is not a dull recitation of a methodology. It is a vigorous and enthusiastic promotion of a research study designed to persuade a funding committee that they must provide support.

Appendix: Questions on study design

The following questions highlight key features of study design which need to be addressed in the protocol. These questions cover the major research methods. They have been adapted, with permission, from *The Pocket Guide to Critical Appraisal* by I.K. Crombie, BMJ Publishing Group, London, 1996.

Designing Surveys

- Is there a description of the population which will be sampled?
- Is there a list of the individuals in the population from which some may be sampled?
- Is the method of sampling described, e.g. simple random, systematic, cluster, stratified?
- Is the method of recruiting study subjects described?
- Is the issue of representativeness addressed?
- Is there a strategy to minimise non-response?
- Is the method of collecting data described, e.g. interview or postal questionnaire?
- Is an outline given of the data items to be collected?
- Is the sample size justified?
- Is there a description of the statistical methods to be used?

Designing Clinical Trials

- Is the patient group described (inclusion and exclusion criteria)?
- Is the method of recruiting study subjects described?
- Is there evidence that the desired number of subjects can be obtained?
- Are there procedures for obtaining informed consent?
- Is the method of randomisation described?
- Is the intervention clearly described?
- Is there a good argument why the intervention should work?
- Is the control treatment clearly described?
- Is the study double blind?
- Is the primary outcome measure clearly defined, clinically relevant, likely to be accurately measured?
- Is account taken of other factors which could influence the outcome?
- Is there a strategy to minimise losses to follow up?
- Is the sample size justified?
- Is there a description of the statistical methods to be used?

Designing Cohort Studies

- Is the study group clearly defined?
- Is the method of identifying and recruiting subjects described?
- Is the method of follow up described?

- Is the length of follow up justified?
- Is there a strategy to minimise losses to follow up?
- Is the outcome measure clearly defined, clinically relevant, likely to be accurately measured?
- Is account taken of other factors which could influence the outcome?
- Is the sample size justified?
- Is there evidence that the desired number of subjects can be obtained?
- Is there a description of the statistical methods to be used?

Designing Case Control Studies

- Are the cases clearly defined?
- Do the controls come from the same general population as the cases?
- Are the methods of recruiting cases and controls described?
- Is the method of collecting data described, e.g. interview or postal questionnaire?
- Will data be collected in the same way for cases and controls?
- Is the sample size justified?
- Is there evidence that the desired number of cases and controls can be obtained?
- Is there a description of the statistical methods to be used?

Designing Qualitative Studies

- Is the theoretical basis of the study described?
- Is the method of data collection described?
- Is the role of the researcher discussed?
- Is it clear how the analysis will be performed?
- Does the person who will conduct the analysis have sufficient experience?

Designing Economic Evaluation

- Is an economist mentioned in the proposal?
- Is the relevant economic theory described?
- Is the method of costing described?
- Is the source of costing data identified?
- Is the health outcome measure described?

Books on research and critical appraisal

Bailey, D. M. *Research for the Health Professional. A Practical Guide.* F.A. Davies, Philadelphia, 1991.

Crombie, I.K. *The Pocket Guide to Critical Appraisal.* BMJ Publishing Group, London, 1996.

Crombie, I.K. and Davies, H.T.O. *Research in Health Care: The Design, Conduct and Interpretation of Health Services Research.* J. Wiley, Chichester, 1996.

Hulley, S. B. and Cummings, S. R. (eds). *Designing Clinical Research.* Williams and Wilkins, Baltimore, 1988.

Chapter 7 Common failings

Grant applications resemble snowflakes in that no two are ever alike (they are also similar in having rather short life expectancies). Despite their diversity, there is a relatively small number of reasons why some applications are not funded. This chapter reviews those reasons.

Uninspiring project

One of the hazards of seeking research support is that projects which are important to the applicants may be thought dull by the funding committee. Projects which are most important are those whose findings will have national or, better, international implications. Dull projects will include those which, although they may be important locally, have little national relevance. These include projects which describe the types of patients who attend a local clinic or which identify the difficulties of providing services to a particular community. Such projects will not be candidates for funding unless it is clear that general lessons can be learned from local circumstances.

A separate category of uninspiring projects are those which propose to collect masses of data without indicating what ideas will be tested and what new knowledge gained. Even national surveys will be judged as poor if there is not a clear statement of how the data will be used. Funding bodies are not impressed by proposals to collect the data now and do the thinking later. They prefer a clear statement of the aims, which indicates precisely how the study will contribute to our understanding.

The final category of dull project is one in which answers to the research questions are largely known. Applicants sometimes appear not to have reviewed the literature properly. This can occur when studies are published in types of journals which the applicants do not commonly read. There is no alternative to careful computerised literature searches using databases such as Medline, EMBase, and Psychlit.

Overambitious project

At the opposite end of the scale from dull projects are those which, if successful, would completely revolutionise the delivery of health care. It might be thought that a really ambitious project, which would have major implications, would be irresistible to funding bodies. The problem lies in the qualification, the need for success. In general the more ambitious a project, the more likely it will fail.

Overambition can creep in when projects have many different aims. Experienced researchers know how difficult it is to carry out even simple studies successfully and consider the pursuit of several aims simultaneously to be a recipe for disaster. Similarly, projects which promise major changes, for example in disease outcome or in professional behaviour, are viewed with scepticism. Some research studies may provide evidence of a modest improvement in health care, but seldom are larger changes achieved.

These cautions do not mean that groundbreaking research will never be funded. If you can demonstrate that you have a feasible method and the necessary experience to carry out a complex study, then it may be funded. Similarly, if you can provide good research evidence to show why you expect major improvements in disease outcome, then your application will be carefully considered. However, it is much more difficult to make a good case for a complex study than for a simple one. Unless you are very confident of being able to do so, select a project which combines modest aims with clever ideas.

Rambling description

Some grant applications read as if they had been translated from Greek by a scholar whose linguistic skills were restricted to Sanskrit. The study methods may be introduced, briefly abandoned for a discourse on statistical techniques, before being expanded upon with gusto. The explanation for the confusion is often that the study design has evolved gradually and the emerging complexities are laid out in the sequence in which the applicants dealt with them.

It is difficult to write a concise, clear description of a proposed study. Research can be a complex business, with a host of issues to be taken into account. Unless these are marshalled in a logical sequence, reviewers may misunderstand and wrongly label the project as flawed. This is unfortunate, but the responsibility for producing a clear, readable account lies with the applicants.

Poorly developed methodology

Research proposals sometimes present an interesting question but do not explain how research will be conducted. Instead, some unhelpful statement may be made such as: "A survey will be done" or "A questionnaire will be developed". These statements immediately raise questions about what exactly will be done, how it will be done, and what data items will be collected. Equally vague phrases are: "A number of staff will be interviewed" (what types of staff and how many?); "Clinical characteristics will be recorded" (which ones?); "Patient progress will be monitored" (which features and for how long?); "High risk patients will be identified" (how?). Omitting these details conveys the impression that the study has not been properly thought through.

The problem of poorly developed methodology can easily be overcome by reviewing the protocol, asking whether each detail is properly defined and fully explained. Being precise need not lengthen the protocol. For example, it takes less space to say "50 senior nurses" than it does to say "a number of nurses", yet the difference in the impression of the thoroughness of the design is huge.

An excess of clinical detail

Research studies which focus on the outcome of particular treatments inevitably involve some clinical description. This will cover the signs and symptoms used in diagnosis and the rationale

43

for the treatments given as well as clinical features used in assessing the outcomes. Health professionals are well aware of the many subtle variations between patients that can influence both choice of treatment and outcome. There is a strong temptation to include this information in the applications so that it is swamped with excessive clinical detail. These factors are important for the management of individual patients but they are usually not needed in the grant application. Instead, the application should be pruned of unnecessary elaboration. If you cannot bear to lose these details altogether, consign them to an appendix (which will probably not be read by a hard pressed reviewer). The research design needs to stand clear, unencumbered by clinical niceties.

Insufficient expertise

Research in health care is often multidisciplinary. For example, with the growing pressure on resources, assessment of the costs of the delivery of care is an increasing feature of research studies. Thus, the project could involve an economic appraisal. Further, much of health care is influenced by individual behaviour, be it patient or health professional. Many projects are concerned with changing behaviour and thus move into the realm of health psychology. Multidisciplinary projects are welcomed by funding bodies, in part because the crossfertilisation between disciplines can enrich the research. However, if there is a component of economics, psychology or some other discipline then it is best to have a specialist in that field as a co-applicant. Funding committees do not welcome research where the applicants have no experience in the field.

Conditional projects

Many research projects propose to undertake some preliminary development work before beginning the main study. This may be the preparation of a questionnaire to assess patient satisfaction or the development of a diagnostic algorithm for the early detection of a disease or it could be a pilot study to determine whether sufficient numbers of patients could be recruited to the study. The problem with each of these examples is that if the preliminary work should be unsuccessful the main study cannot proceed. The main study is thus conditional on the first part.

Funding committees are naturally reluctant to fund conditional projects. They do not want to commit £100 000 to learn subsequently that the study foundered because of a failure at an early stage. Their response might be to ask the researchers to show that the conditional stage will work, before giving funding. Possibly they may offer to support the preliminary study, with the promise of further funding should it be successful. The moral here is to avoid conditional projects where possible. Either carry out the development work before submitting or choose a project for which you can provide evidence that all the steps will work.

Cobbled together applications

Some applications read as if they were thrown together in a few days. The literature review may be incomplete or sometimes is totally missing. The study methods are poorly described and there is often repetition. At worst there may be handwritten comments in the manuscript which were meant to be, but were not, incorporated into the text. The overall impression is one of haste, of a lack of attention to detail. Reviewers will lose confidence in the ability of the applicants to complete the study. The most likely consequence is that the funding will not be awarded.

Key lessons

Funding committees rely on the quality of the application as a guide to the likely success of a project. Many grant applications simply do not meet the expectations of funding committees. These applications are often poorly written, the research question may not be clearly expressed, the description of the methods may be inadequate or it may contain serious flaws. Fortunately, there are a number of strategies which can be employed to improve the quality of applications. These are described in the next chapter.

Chapter 8 Strategies for success

Previous chapters have outlined the review process, the criteria on which grant applications are assessed, and the most common failings. It is not too difficult to write a good quality application; the problem is that it is all too easy to write a poor one. This chapter outlines the strategies to follow to ensure your application is of high quality.

Allow enough time

Having decided to prepare a grant application, a compulsion can set in to complete and submit it as quickly as possible. This is often done against a submission deadline of only a few weeks. It is not clear why this panic takes hold. The ideas behind the research have probably been kicking about for several months and there is seldom a reason for sudden urgency. There is a real cost to this rapid action: "Written in haste, rejected at leisure" is a suitable maxim for grant applications. Instead of yielding to non-existent pressures, it is better to allow adequate time to prepare and write a decent application. The time required will vary greatly but if an application is conceived and written within six weeks it will almost certainly be of poor quality. In setting the time, it can be helpful to nominate dates for the completion of first, second, and final drafts to encourage progress with the writing.

There is no fixed rule for the length of time required. Some researchers try to allow at least six months for the whole process. Others feel that six months is too short, requiring a longer period to mature the research ideas and the methods. Whatever the time, it is best to submit only when you are confident the application is of high quality.

Select the funding body with care

The range of funding bodies and the diversity of their interests make careful targeting of grant applications essential. If the wrong funding body has been picked then much effort and time can be wasted. There is no alternative to exploring funding bodies in some detail to establish their preferences for types of topic and even preferred choice of research method.

Follow the instructions

Most funding bodies issue detailed instructions on the completion of grant applications. It may seem unnecessary to advise that these be followed carefully, but such is the case. Many applicants ignore some of the requirements, weakening their application by doing so. Reviewers may feel that if the applicants cannot follow the instructions, they may not be competent to carry out high quality research.

One of the most common breaches is to overrun the stated length of the application. If the instructions say no more than six pages to describe the method, then keep to this. Long applications induce heartsink in reviewers, who may feel that if applicants cannot write to the proper length they may be unable to run a research project. Most applications, especially long ones, can usually be cut by getting rid of unnecessary detail. (The most common example of this is in the background information. Some applications give a blow by blow history of how the project came about, most of which is of no relevance.) It is not enough to reduce the font size or decrease the margins so that more text can be crammed in. This will simply antagonise the reviewer. Instead, take out the red pen and cut with vigour.

Another common problem is the omission of a sample size calculation. This is often requested in instructions which accompany the application form. If it is missed out the application may be sent back with a request to include it. However, if this failing is merely one of several the application may be rejected outright. As it is easy to calculate (see a statistician if you have any problems), it is best to present it.

Begin writing

Committing ideas to paper is often a salutary experience. What may have seemed clear and logical in the mind can prove to be confused and incoherent when written. It is best to get ideas on paper at an early stage, particularly for collaborative ventures. It is all too easy to spend several happy hours discussing a project with colleagues without making real progress. Instead, the main features of the study design should be committed to paper. These include: the aims, the choice of research method, the source and characteristics of the study subjects, and the measurements to be made. The details will seldom be fully worked out when writing begins but the important point about writing is to begin.

Write clearly

The instruction to write clearly is one of those gratuitously offensive remarks with which teachers have alienated students for generations. Nevertheless, examples of poor writing are commonly encountered in grant applications. The purpose of a grant application is not to impress readers with your erudition but to convey your ideas without misunderstanding. If the members of a funding committee cannot understand parts of an application, they are apt to conclude that it is flawed and reject it.

There are several types of common error. Long sentences, with many subclauses, should be avoided. The longer the sentence, the greater the chance that it will cause confusion (a long sentence is one that exceeds 30 words or three lines of text). Pompous phrases (e.g. the relativistic pluripotential of this overarching synthesis) should be deleted. A good practice is to search through the grant application for high flown phrases and translate them into plain English. Technical terms should be carefully checked to ensure the exact meaning is conveyed. Jargon (i.e. terms with which the funding body may not be familiar) should be fully explained. Acronyms and abbreviations are also best avoided: they may make perfect sense to the researcher who has been living with them for many months but are likely to be impenetrable to everyone else. Word processing packages supply spell checking and grammar checking packages which are well worth using.

Write with three reviewers in mind

Grant applications will be assessed by three groups of reviewers and must be written to satisfy all three.

The expert referees will expect the application to be methodologically rigorous and to review all the relevant literature. Thus the study design and the background to the study have to be of a high standard.

The professional secretariat of the funding body will want to be reassured that the project fits with their policy interests. They will also be concerned with the implications of the findings.

Finally, there will be some members of the committee who have little experience of your field of research or of the method to be used. The application has to be written so that it can be easily followed by the non-expert.

Problems sometimes arise because researchers have such a detailed knowledge of their research topic. The ideas underpinning the research, the methodology, and even the technical terms used to describe it may all appear perfectly clear. But it may be opaque to the reviewers. To avoid this, think of the reviewers as intelligent specialists from different disciplines and write with them in mind.

Allowance should also be made for the grant application being read in some haste. Some funding committees are so overburdened that this is inevitable. If this happens some details may be missed and others misunderstood. Thus, the application needs to be written so clearly that it can be easily understood with the most cursory of readings.

Explain why the study will succeed

One of the key issues which concerns funding committees is whether the study will be concluded satisfactorily. This does not mean that you must be able to predict what answer you will get to the research question. There would be little point in doing the research if the answer were obvious. Instead, the application should demonstrate that the study will work in the sense that it will produce data which will provide a meaningful answer to the research question. To do this, you must show that the project has a sound theoretical basis, that there is an important question to be answered, and that the chosen research design is the best way to answer it. The issue of feasibility should also be addressed to show that the study subjects can be identified and a sufficient number recruited, and that the data collection process will be successful. Finally, you must describe the statistical techniques which will be used.

Seek advice

It is essential to obtain comments on a grant application from individuals who can bring a fresh eye to the text. There are several sources of comment. Most funding bodies welcome early contact from potential applicants. It is the job of funding bodies to give out monies and they try to organise their procedures to encourage high quality applications. They are happy to advise whether the topic is one in which they are likely to be interested. They will indicate whether the level and type of support fit their funding strategy. Most will also take the time to provide constructive comments on research proposals. These should be graciously acknowledged and incorporated whenever possible. It is acceptable to disagree with a few, giving powerful arguments for doing so. The comments should never be ignored, as this will only offend.

Colleagues can provide help in a variety of ways. They can act as a sounding board for ideas. They may come up with suggestions and, if not, the process of explaining your ideas can help clarify them in your own mind. Colleagues can also be useful in assessing the readability of the grant application. If there is a part which they cannot follow, there is every likelihood the reviewers will have the same difficulty. Thus when misunderstandings are identified do not blame your colleague, rewrite the protocol.

Review the layout

Layout is a key feature of the grant application. The overall appearance matters because your application will be one among 20 or 30 others. If it doesn't look professional it will be subconsciously marked down.

A key feature of layout is the contribution it makes to ease of understanding. The careful use of headings and subheadings provides the reader with a map of the application, showing where each section fits in with the whole. The headings should be marked by the judicious use of font type, font size, italics or bold type. If a series of points is being made or a set of data items is being listed, these could be presented as bullet points. The use of these features can enliven an application. There is little more offputting than page after page of unrelieved text.

Attention to layout is important because it is easy to get lost when reading a grant. Questions which commonly arise in the mind of the reviewer are: Why am I being given this information? How does it fit in with the rest of the application? These questions, and the censure which they imply, can be avoided through the judicious use of subheadings. If this is not done then pieces of information which are essential to the application may be missed because the reader was puzzled about their value. (Many researchers have had grant applications rejected not because the protocol was flawed, but because points of detail in the text were missed by the reviewer. It is tempting to blame the reviewer for being half blind and illiterate, but the fault lies with the writer.)

Keep trying

When you have submitted the application, do not be too optimistic; it is best to expect some refusals. This is a counsel not of despair but of realism. Grant applications have a very high rejection rate. Many funding bodies reject over two thirds of the applications they receive. Some researchers reckon that a lifetime success rate of one in three is good going. Others say that when starting out, their success rate was low but as experience accumulated, success became more common.

Knowing that you will not always be successful in submissions has important consequences. Firstly, it will help soften the blow if your application is rejected. More importantly, this knowledge provides some motivation to prepare an application of good enough quality to be funded.

If you are unsuccessful don't just discard the application, think where else you could send it. Funding bodies are very varied and what is rejected by one may appeal to another. Take advantage of any feedback received on the application, modify it accordingly, and submit it to another agency. Most researchers have experience of an application which was turned down by one body only to be funded by another.

Key lessons

One feature of success, whatever the field of activity, is that it is unfairly distributed. Some people gain what seems an undue share whilst others, who would seem to merit much, receive little. Grant applications need to be drafted carefully to ensure that they are easily followed and that the implications of the research are appreciated. They need to be written to satisfy the expert reviewer whilst being accessible to the non-specialist members of the committee. The writer may find it hard to identify sections which are confusing or difficult to follow. One approach is to put the application to one side for a few weeks so that it can be taken up again with a fresh mind. Many will find they do not have time for this. An alternative is to ask one or more colleagues who are unfamiliar with the project to read it. If there are parts which cause difficulty do not blame the colleague, rewrite the text. Seeking advice from others greatly increases the chances of funding.

Chapter 9 Writing the detailed application

Although funding sources may be diverse, most grant applications follow a broadly similar pattern. A single chapter can readily address the requirements of almost all funding bodies. This chapter reviews in turn the sections of the grant application, giving advice on each.

Title

The title is the first part of the application to be read. It is the one in which most information is conveyed in fewest words. It indicates the broad area of research, introduces the research question, and may also specify the research method to be used. (The uninformative phrase "a study of" should be avoided in favour of naming the appropriate research design, e.g. "a survey" or "a randomised controlled trial".) The most important requirement is that the main purpose or the principal research question should be stated briefly. The title should be short, in general no more than 12–15 words. The title requires much more effort, per word, than any other section of the application.

Summary

Many, but not all, application forms request a short summary of the protocol. This presents the key parts of the application in miniature. As with the title, the summary needs to be carefully composed. It provides a map of the whole application so that the reader knows what to expect and understands how each part of the application relates to the others. Depending on the funding body, the summary may range from 100 to 400 words. Sometimes the word length is not stated and the applicant is given a fixed space in which to write. It is better to use fewer than more words. Do not cram extra text (e.g. single spaced font size 8) into a small space. This will antagonise reviewers and encourage them to skim through the abstract. In contrast, a spaciously laid out brief summary will invite close attention. Methodological detail should be avoided; the summary gives an overview of the project, not the technicalities of the study.

The layout of a typical summary of, say, 150 words (assuming sentences of 15–18 words) is as follows.

- It should introduce the topic, explaining why more research is needed (in one or two sentences).
- Then it should state the main aim of the research, expanding on the information given in the title (one sentence).
- Brief details of the study method should follow, including the chosen research design, the nature and number of the study subjects, and the broad categories of data to be collected (two to three sentences).
- Finally, it should indicate what the main findings would be and the implications which flow from these (one to two sentences).

With this layout the whole summary will come well within the permitted maximum length, allowing a clear, attractive presentation.

Supervision

Many application forms ask how many hours per week the applicants intend to spend supervising the project. This section is easy to complete, requiring only the insertion of a number, but the answers are carefully assessed. If all the applicants state they will donate one hour per week to the project, funding is unlikely. The day to day supervision can amount to 6–8 hours per week and someone has to take responsibility for it. Usually the lead applicant will undertake the major part of this, with the other applicants supplying 1–2 hours per week. However, if one of the applicants has a particular skill which is central to the project, then that person should volunteer more than this minimum contribution.

Ethical permission

Medical research is often intrusive. Even the simple act of sending a questionnaire can be upsetting; subjects may wonder why they were selected, whether this means they are at special risk of becoming ill. Thus in all but a few exceptional circumstances, funding for medical research will only be awarded if ethical permission is obtained. This is decided by the local research ethics committees located in each health authority. These meet regularly, often once per month, to consider proposed studies. For multicentre projects which involve five or more individual local research ethics committees, researchers can apply to a multicentre research ethics committee. These have been set up in each of the English regions and in Scotland and Wales, to streamline the applications procedure.

The main ethical concerns are whether the research will place the subjects under undue risk and whether the subjects are fully informed about the nature of the study. The ethics committee will review the study documentation, including the procedures to obtain informed consent. If approved, the committee will send a formal letter which should be enclosed with the grant application.

Background (Introduction)

Many application forms ask for a section on background to the research. Do not be misled by this term. It is not asking for details of the personal odyssey which led to the application being developed. Instead, it is seeking the scientific background to the research question. The background section often begins with a statement of the importance of the research area, e.g. the number of people who suffer from the disease being studied, or the cost that it presents to the NHS. It should provide a brief review of the landmark studies as well as the recent ones. (If you omit the recent studies it will be assumed that you are not up to date with the literature.)

This background is not intended to present an exhaustive review of present knowledge. Rather it should be making the case for the need for further research by establishing the importance of the topic and highlighting the gaps in our present knowledge. The background often concludes with the broad long term goals of the proposed research.

Aims

The aims should provide a succinct statement of what the project intends to find out. Fishing expeditions, undertaken in the hope that something might turn up, are rarely funded. Committees take the view that if the applicants are not sure what they are looking for, they are unlikely to find anything. Some funding bodies ask for the aims to be stated as hypotheses to be tested, others as research questions to be answered. Usually three or four aims should be listed as too many aims give the impression of an overambitious project. The aims do not offer a description of the research methods or of the data which will be collected. They are concerned with the purposes of the research, not the means.

A lucid statement of the aims can be difficult to achieve. When first conceived, research ideas can appear attractive, even exciting. More mature assessment can reveal that the idea was poorly thought out: it may hold the glimmer of a good idea like a flake of gold in a lump of rock. The original concept may be too ambitious (e.g. involving many different groups of subjects) or too difficult to study (e.g. requiring an accuracy of measurement which is unattainable). It could involve substantially more subjects than could be reasonably recruited or it might require cooperation from professionals who have little interest in the topic. There are many reasons why the first outline of a research idea may be poor. All researchers have to clarify the aims to make sure they are attainable and that they are worth attaining.

Plan of the investigation

The plan of the investigation presents the research design in detail. It is by far the longest section of the application, often running to four or five pages. The challenge is to provide sufficient information to be convincing without drowning the reader in an excess of technical detail. To achieve this the plan should be divided into several subsections. These orientate readers and lead them through the steps of the study design. The following subsections should, with minor modifications, be suitable for most funding bodies.

Overview

Providing a brief overview of the study design prepares the reader for what is to come. This should state the research method to be used (e.g. cross-sectional survey, case control study or clinical trial). It should indicate briefly who will be studied and how the requisite data will be obtained. All of these topics should then be expanded upon later.

Study subjects

The study subjects, be they patients or health professionals, need to be described in detail. The criteria used to select them (e.g. age range or gender) should be given. When diagnostic criteria have been used to define a patient group, these should also be stated, together with criteria which would be used to exclude some from investigation (e.g. too severely ill, presence of other disease, too old or too young). The process by which study subjects will be recruited should also be given. This could be done in a number of ways: from clinic lists, from GP case notes, from computerised patient lists. The key points are to demonstrate that the subjects can be identified and a sufficient number recruited.

Data to be collected

The types of data to be collected should be listed, indicating how each item will be measured. If either a postal questionnaire or an interview is to be used, a list of the items to be covered should be given. It is not necessary to have the completed proforma but nor is it enough to say that a questionnaire will be developed. Sufficient detail must be presented to demonstrate that considerable thought has been given to what will be collected. If physical measurements are to be made (e.g. peak flow or blood pressure) the type of equipment which will be used should be described. Finally, if biochemical factors are to be measured (e.g. serum cholesterol, urinary sodium or salivary cotinine) the analytical techniques to be used should be described. In many instances a published paper will give the methodological details and it may be sufficient to cite

THE POCKET GUIDE TO GRANT APPLICATIONS

that. In other cases a fuller description will be required. The description of the data collection process should demonstrate that accurate reliable data will be obtained.

Study procedures

The logistics of research studies often need careful planning. Funding committees want to know that the following sorts of questions have been addressed and answered.

- How will subjects be identified and contacted?
- What sampling methods will be used?
- Where will subjects be interviewed?
- How will the interviews be organised?
- Who will carry out the interviews?
- How will the interviewers be trained?

Some studies involve following patients over time; the protocol should describe how followup contacts will be organised. In addition, for randomised controlled trials, the method of randomisation and the strategies to preserve blinding will have to be given. The funding committee want reassurance that all of the study procedures will be carried out successfully.

Data analysis

A limited description is needed of the statistical techniques to be used. It is usually sufficient to mention a few techniques, such as chi squared tests, multiple regression or Cox proportional hazards. The appropriate statistical techniques are usually clear from the study design and the specification of the data to be collected. All funding committees will include a professional statistician who will check these details. If you are unsure which statistical procedures to use then seek advice from a statistician. Further, if the statistical analysis is likely to be extensive, it might be best to have a statistician as a co-applicant. This will persuade the committee that you have the necessary expertise on the team.

Sample size calculation

Formal sample size calculations are now a requirement for all research studies. These indicate how many study subjects are required so that, if the research ideas prove correct, a statistically significant result will be obtained. If the study is too small a real effect may be overlooked. If it is too large then resources will be wasted. Some researchers are confident about performing their own sample size calculations. Others prefer to engage a statistician. However they are performed, the calculations need to be a prominent part of the application.

References

The references should be cited in the text using one of the standard conventions. The most common is the Vancouver style in which references are cited in the text using sequential numbers and listed in numerical order in the reference list. This style minimises the space required in the text, an advantage as space is usually at a premium. Details of this style are printed each year in the first issue of the *British Medical Journal*.

Timetable of work

The conduct of the study usually falls into three main sections. The initial period will involve piloting and finalising the study procedures. This phase may take between one and three months, usually accounting for less than 10% of the overall time. It is followed by the identification and recruitment of the study subjects and the collection of the data. This stage takes the longest time, commonly ranging from nine months to two and a half years. The length of time should realistically reflect the number of subjects to be recruited and the method of data collection. Finally, there is a period for analysis of the data and the preparation of the final report and papers for publication. This often takes between two and six months.

The information on the timings should be presented as a table or a flow diagram indicating the activity and the amount of time, in months, that it will take. The detail given need not be great unless the study design is particularly complex. But it should identify the stage at which the major milestones (e.g. patient recruitment, completion of interviews, processing and analysis of data) will be completed. The main purpose of the timetable is to indicate how the overall time of the study will be allocated. This enables the funding committee to check that sufficient time has been allocated to each stage.

Existing facilities

Funding bodies like to feel that they are getting good value for money, an impression fostered if some of the necessary facilities are being provided by the applicants. It is usually expected that office space and furniture will be supplied. But there can be an advantage in declaring some additional facilities where possible. These might include specialised equipment that you already have such as computer software or hardware. Alternatively, the host institution may be willing to provide a small amount of secretarial support. It is not necessary to make a sizable contribution to the study, it is just to give the impression that the applicant is not seeking every single item down to the last pencil and rubber.

Justification of costs

Funding bodies will meet all reasonable costs encountered during the conduct of a research study. However, you must point out why the specified costs are reasonable. For example, it may be clear to the applicants why their study needs a research assistant for three years and a part time secretary as well. But the committee, who have given far less thought to the detailed mechanics of the study, will not be impressed unless an adequate explanation is given for each of the costs. Thus for each person to be employed, there should be a brief but explicit statement of their tasks. If an experienced, and hence expensive, person is to be employed then the reason why special skills are needed should be given. If a computer is requested then some explanation is needed of the uses which will be made of it (e.g. drafting letters and questionnaires, analysis of data). If travel expenses are claimed details of the number and the average length of the trips should be stated. It is usually not necessary to justify minor items, such as £50 on postage, but all costly items, certainly anything more than £300, should be justified.

Purpose and potential

Most application forms have a section in which the researchers can explain the impact the study findings will have on health care delivery. If there is no heading provided then insert one, as this section provides vital information. It informs the funding body what they will get for their money. It is essential that they get as much as possible.

Many researchers fail to explain why their project deserves to be funded. This can be a consequence of overfamiliarity with the research ideas. You may feel that it is self-evident that the topic is crucial and needs funding. However, this rationale needs to be given on paper. As funding bodies want to support important research, it is essential to demonstrate that your project falls into this category. Explain what the results will do for patient care or how they will improve it or save money. Clarify how the implications are not limited to the narrow confines of the project, but will carry across to much wider areas of health care. It is no use hoping that the funding body will appreciate the worth of a study. The application must make an irresistible case for funding.

Curricula vitae

A brief CV of each applicant should be submitted with the application. It will give the name, age, qualifications (degrees and diplomas), current post, and recent publications. The CV is checked to ensure that the applicants have sufficient experience and the relevant skills (e.g. clinical, statistical or research design). Thus it should be written to demonstrate the necessary expertise. When listing your degrees, give details of the subject when this is relevant to the project. Similarly, the description of your current post should clarify both seniority and area of expertise. Finally, the recent publications should, if possible, be in the same field as the proposed study. It is best to use publications in peer reviewed journals: conference presentations and meeting abstracts carry little weight.

A final check

Grant applications evolve as they are being written; the aims may change and certainly the research design will be refined as the details are gradually worked out. In some cases this can result in a disjointed application. The background, which should introduce the aims, may not do so in the final version. In turn the research design may no longer fit closely with the study aims. Make sure there is consistency between background, aims, methods, purpose, and potential. Check that the data to be collected will answer the research questions and that the study subjects can be recruited. Examine the layout to make sure the application is easy to follow. Finally, run the spellcheck to get rid of the last few typos.

Chapter 10 A computer based aid to writing grants

When writing the text of a grant application, applicants may want to check some of the detailed advice given in this book. However, the book may not be to hand or it may prove difficult to locate the desired information. To assist the preparation of applications, we have prepared a computer based aid.

Layout of the computer based aid

The computer based aid is designed to sit at the side of the computer screen while you type your protocol. The word processor occupies the remainder, and the major part, of the screen. To be of most use, the aid is organised in the sections into which grant applications are usually divided. These are:

- title
- summary
- introduction
- aims
- plan
- sample size
- purpose and potential of the results
- ethics
- timetable
- existing facilities
- financial plan
- justification of requirements
- references
- supervision
- curricula vitae.

You can call up advice on each section by clicking on the relevant button. The program provides an on screen *aide memoire* of key points and includes practical explanations of how to complete an application.

The plan

By far the largest of the sections of the computer based aid is the plan. It presents the research design in detail and comprises the following sections:

- overview
- study design
- study subjects
- data to be collected
- study procedures
- data analysis.

When the plan button is clicked, a further menu listing the component sections is shown.

Help menu bar

There is a help file which can be opened by clicking on Help on the menu bar and then selecting Contents. It describes how to use the package and how to navigate through it. It lists the program's buttons and outlines their functions. It also describes the other menus which are available within the package. It is there to help you the first time you open the program and at other times if you get stuck.

Installation

The program runs on IBM compatible PCs under Windows 3.1, Windows 95 or Windows NT. It has been designed for a screen resolution of 800×600 pixels or higher, although most of it is useable at a resolution of 640×480.

Place the disk in your floppy disk drive. Open File Manager, display the list of files on the floppy drive (usually drive A:) and double click on the file name Setup.exe. In Windows 95 or NT use the Add/Remove Programs facility on the control panel. Follow the instructions on your screen. To start the program, double click the Grant program icon in the Grant program group. The program has a number of facilities, including the way the advice is displayed and help with sample size estimations. To take full advantage of the program, be sure to read the help (click Help and Contents on the menu bar).

Other learning aids

If you work in a UK higher education institute, you should have free access to a computer assisted learning package entitled Studying Populations. It was designed and written by a team of researchers and teachers including the authors of this book. The program teaches about methods used in health services research and has many interactive exercises on study design and sampling. It may help you understand the issues surrounding good study design and improve your confidence in writing applications. If your institution does not have the package, contact Dr JD Baty by email at JDBaty@dundee.ac.uk.

Index